WHAT TO EAT WITH POTS

Using Whole Foods to Relieve Postural Orthostatic Tachycardia Syndrome

Rose Annear

CONTENTS

Introduction

POTS or postural orthostatic tachycardia syndrome is a circulatory disorder that causes a number of symptoms when a person transitions from lying down to standing up, such as lightheadedness, rapid heartbeat, fatigue or a drop in blood pressure.

This condition affects about 1-3 million people in the US alone. Interestingly, women make up a large percentage of this number, typically between the age of 15 and 60.

The reason why a person with POTS may feel faint, dizzy or lightheaded is because the condition causes less blood to return to the heart after they change position. Although symptoms usually improve as one gets older, changing diet can greatly help to ease them, especially with regards to the severity and how frequent they occur.

Luckily, POTS usually resolves on its own.

This book contains the essential information you need if you're looking for a nutritional guide for POTS. It answers questions such as what a POTS diet should look like, some modifications and lifestyle interventions that can help you on your road to recovery. More importantly, I have included several recipes to help you get started.

What Is POTS?

Before we delve into the diet plan, let's start with the basics. So, what is POTS?

POTS, which stands for postural orthostatic tachycardia syndrome, is a form of dysautonomia that tends to affect blood flow, leading to dizziness when you stand.

Before we proceed, let's break down the acronym POTS, as I believe it will help us grasp the full meaning of this condition.

Postural: As the name suggests, this has to do with the posture or position of the body. People with POTS normally experience associated symptoms when they try to change their position.

Orthostatic: This is a form of blood pressure drop that causes dizziness. Normally, it is how your body responds when you sit, stand, or change your position. The pressure drop happens as you change from one position to another, such as when you stand up from a sitting/lying position.

Tachycardia: This is a clinical term used to describe a fast heart rate, usually above 100 beats per minute. In patients with POTS, there's an increased heart rate due to the dysregulation of their autonomic system. So, the blood pressure is anything but normal.

Syndrome: This refers to a group of symptoms that tend to occur together in patients. It doesn't necessarily mean it's a disease.

Having simplified the terms, we can now take a step further without sounding too "technical." We can now describe POTS as a neurological disorder that occurs when the nervous system doesn't respond normally, usually to changes in the position of the body. Talking about the nervous system, we are interested in the autonomic nervous function.

The autonomic nervous system is responsible for a lot of involuntary actions such as digestion, heartbeat, getting sexually aroused, balance and so on. Also, when you stand, it is the autonomic function that ensures the appropriate amount of blood gets to the upper body.

Generally, POTS is more experienced in adult women, usually from the age of 15 to 50. In most cases, the cause is not clear. It is often noticed during pregnancy; other triggers are surgery, a virus infection or vaccination. In fact, it is reported that up to 2-14 percent COVID patients develop POTS.

As earlier indicated, POTS patients usually have an increased heart rate. This can be an increase of 30 beats per minute or over 120 beats per minute after the person stands for 10 minutes.

Types of POTS

Like many other conditions, POTS come in different types; although the origin might not always be known. Let's quickly look at the more common ones.

Hypovolemic POTS

As the name suggests, this type of POTS is usually associated with hypovolemic patients. hypovolemia, a condition where a person suffers a rapid loss of fluids or blood from their body.

Neuropathic POTS

This type of POTS occurs when a person's nerves are damaged and as a result restricts blood flow from the legs to the heart.

The affected nerves in question are often regarded as small fiber nerves and are responsible for blood vessel constriction in the limbs and abdomen.

Hyperandrenegic POTS

As the name suggests, this type of POTS occurs with people that have a high level of norepinephrine or stress hormone.

Secondary POTS

POTS can also be secondary if it occurs as a result of an underlying condition or disease that is linked to autonomic neuropathy, which can lead to dysautonomia. This includes autoimmune diseases like lupus and Sjogren's syndrome or diabetes.

Common Causes & Triggers of POTS

There are several causes of POTS. Just like the types, we can categorize these into primary and secondary causes.

Primary causes are those that are the underlying source of the condition in a patient. These include but not limited to viruses, neuropathy, nitric oxide, and so on.

Secondary causes, on the other hand, are when the disease is caused by another condition or disease. Below, you will find some examples:

- Adrenal disorder
- Tumour
- Lyme disease
- Anaemia
- Nutrient deficiencies
- Epstein Barr virus
- Ehlers Danlos syndrome
- Autoimmune disease
- Diabetes

- Deconditioning
- Etc.

In general, the root cause in most cases of POTS is not well understood.

Common Triggers of POTS

In addition to the causes mentioned above, these are also certain conditions and lifestyles that can aggravate the disease. Some of these include:

- Overheating
- Consuming white bread or other refined carbs
- Dehydration
- Pregnancy
- Trauma
- Resting a lot
- Exercise
- Surgery
- Menstrual period

Common Signs You Have POTS

There are certain signs or symptoms that are associated with POTS. However, while these symptoms exist, it doesn't replace the need to get proper diagnosis.

You can only begin the journey to recovery when you know the exact cause of a condition.

People with POTS will often feel dizzy when they stand. Some may even faint when they try to stand. That is why you will often hear POTS being referred to as "the fainting disease". That said, these are just a few of many other symptoms a POT patient may experience.

Below is a list of other signs you can look out for.

- Weakness of the muscle
- Nausea
- Headache
- Fatigue
- Heart palpitations
- General chronic pain
- Abdominal pain

- Chest pain
- Shortness of breath
- Blurred vision
- Insomnia
- Brain fog
- Sweating abnormally
- Bladder dysfunction
- Tremors

Nutrition and Treatment of POTS

When it comes to treating POTS, most treatment plans focus on three main areas - food, lifestyle and medication. Since I'm a strong advocate of naturopathy, I would rather focus on food and lifestyle.

The best diet for POTS is one that is rich in sodium and low in gluten and carb. This has proven to be very effective in many patients.

Having said that, it's also important you exclude certain items from your diet that can hamper your progress.

Talking about lifestyle, exercise is one area not to overlook; don't worry, we will get into that later.

For now, I want us to delve deeper into what a POT diet should look like for you.

The Best POTS Diet for Beginners

As earlier indicated, when dealing with POTS, you want to increase your salt and fluid intake while reducing carbs.

So, why should you go low on carbs?

Well, it's because a carb-filled can actually make your orthostatic symptoms worse. This is because a high carb diet can lower your blood pressure which can be a big problem.

So, the recommendation is to go low on carbs, which is why a keto diet tends to stand out.

A ketogenic diet is low-carb and high-fat. It focuses on greatly reducing carb intake, which changes how the body uses food for fuel or energy by altering your metabolism. In the end, this helps to manage POTS symptoms better and aid recovery in the long run.

Having said that, the categories of foods below are considered to be great for POTS:

- Healthy, salty foods such as pickles and nuts
- High protein foods such as soy, beans and lentils , and white-fleshed fish.
- Whole grains such as brown rice
- Probiotic and probiotic foods

Foods to avoid

- Sweets and sugary foods
- Simple carbs such as white rice, white bread
- Chips
- Pretzels
- Baked goods
- Soda and other sugary drinks

Additional Dietary Tips for POTS

With POTS, anything you can do to alleviate symptoms and raise blood pressure can be helpful. With this mind, here are some dietary tips you should consider.

NB: I have already mentioned some of these, but I would like to go through them again in more detail.

Avoid dehydration

As earlier indicated, staying hydrated is very important for POTS as the condition can make you more sensitive to dehydration.

So, drinking enough water and fluids is highly recommended.

Besides preventing dehydration, this also helps ensure blood is flowing to the head, which eases dizziness.

Even healthy people who drink a lot of water are able to stand for longer periods, and are less likely to faint from standing for so long.

While the amount of water one can drink depends on their size, and level of activity, and weather condition, you should aim to drink up to two liters of water or more per day.

In some cases, it could be less; just make sure you drink enough to maintain a clear urine and prevent dehydration.

Have some salt

Most of the time, people are advised to reduce their salt intake, which is understandable since excess salt is often linked to a number of health problems.

However, for people with POT, having more salt is usually recommended to help increase the blood pressure. In fact, in most cases, the first course of treatment is increasing salt intake.

That said, the type of salt does matter. Personally, I find sea salt more beneficial for POTS but that doesn't mean you can't use table salt. In fact, both types of salt are said to contain comparable amounts of sodium by weight.

You can consume anywhere from 2 to 10 h of salt per day.

Besides cooking, other ways to increase your daily salt intake include taking salt tablets and adding a pinch of salt to your water bottle.

You can also consider some salty snacks such as cheese, miso, smoked fish, olives, pickles, salted nuts and seeds, anchovies, and popcorn (without sugar).

Eat smaller, more frequent meals

Consuming large meals is another thing that can trigger POT symptoms. This is because when a big meal is eaten, the blood diverts blood to aid the digestion process.

In other words, there's increased blood flow to the digestive system.

In addition, eating big meals can make you sleepy.

So, instead of eating a three big meals daily, you can divide it into six smaller meals throughout the day.

This will help ease your POT symptoms and increase your fluid intake.

Sample Whole Food Recipes for POTS

HEMPSEED MILK

Ingredients

- Hempseed (one cup)
- Water (about four cups)
- Coconut oil (1 tbsp.)
- Maple syrup (2 tbsp., can be substituted with coconut nectar)
- Vanilla bean powder (1 tsp., can be substituted with ½ tsp vanilla extract)
- Cinnamon (1 tsp.)

Instructions

1. Put all the ingredients in a blender and blend until it's smooth. This should take a minute or two.

LETTUCE WRAPS

Ingredients

- Two curly kale leaves
- Mayonnaise (1 tbsp.)
- Cooked bacon (four slices)
- One avocado (should be sliced and pitted)
- Four turkey slices (can be swapped with roast chicken)

Instructions

1. Get a cutting board and lay the kale leaves on top. Brush each leaf with your mayonnaise.
2. Now, layer half avocado slice, 2 pieces of bacon and 2 turkey slices on half of each leaf.
3. Roll up each leaf beginning with the end that is filled. Serve! You can keep some in the fridge and reheat when needed.

BERRY BREAKFAST SHAKE

Ingredients

- Half a teaspoon of lemon juice, freshly squeezed
- ¼ cup of mixed berries, frozen
- Half a cup of almond milk or coconut milk
- Half a cup of heavy cream
- One tablespoon of MCT oil (optional)
- One tablespoon of almond butter

Instructions

1. Add all the ingredients to a blender and blend until you get a smooth consistency. Serve immediately.

PECAN, COCONUT & OATMEAL

Ingredients

- Half a cup of coconut or almond milk
- One tablespoon of coconut flakes
- ¼ teaspoon of pure vanilla extract
- ¼ teaspoon of ground cinnamon
- Two tablespoons of almond flour
- Two tablespoons of hemp hearts
- Two teaspoons of chia seeds
- One tablespoon of flax meal
- One tablespoon of pecans, toasted and chopped

Instructions

1. Combine the chia seeds, flax meal, almond flour, cinnamon, vanilla, hemp hearts, and milk in a small pot. Cook over low heat, stirring occasionally until the mixture becomes thick. This should take about 5 minutes.
2. Spoon everything into a bowl or dish and top with coconut flakes and pecans. Serve immediately.

GREEN AVOCADO SMOOTHIE

Ingredients

- Half a cup of spring water
- Two tablespoons of sea moss gel
- One fresh avocado
- One organic burro banana
- Natural sweetener (optional, example is stevia)

Instructions

1. Start by peeling the banana and avocado.
2. Add to a blender together with the sea moss gel, sweetener, and water. Blend until smooth.

TASTY PANINI

Ingredients

- One ripe banana, chopped
- Two slices whole grain bread
- ¼ cup natural peanut butter
- ¼ cup hot water
- ¼ cup raisin
- 1 tsp cinnamon
- 2 tsp cacao powder

Instructions

1. In a bowl, combine the hot water, cinnamon, and cacao powder. Mix well.
2. Next, spread the butter on the bread slices.
3. Place the chopped bananas on the toast.
4. Now, combine the raisin and mixture from step 1 in a blender and spread it on the sandwich.

ROASTED TOMATO AND BELL PEPPER SOUP

Ingredients

- Five tomatoes (choose large ones)
- Three large red bell pepper (quartered, seeded)
- 4-6 garlic cloves (peeled)
- Olive oil (two teaspoons)
- Thyme (one teaspoon, fresh & minced)
- Fresh minced basil (two tablespoons)
- Vegetable stock (two cups, make sure it's low in fat and sodium)
- Salt & pepper to taste

Directions

1. Start by preheating the oven. Set it to 450 degrees Fahrenheit.
2. Get an oiled baking sheet. Place the peppers, garlic, and tomatoes on the sheet.

3. Next, drizzle olive oil over the vegetables and roast for half an hour or until they become brownish.

4. Take the vegetables out from the oven and let it cool. Then puree them in a blender.

5. Next transfer the pureed vegetables to a saucepan, then add your thyme and stock and bring to soup consistency.

6. Now, pour in the basil and boil. Use medium heat.

7. The soup is best served cold!

QUINOA PORRIDGE

Ingredients

- ½ cup coconut milk or cream
- 1 cup dry quinoa
- ½ tsp cayenne
- ½ lime, with skin grated
- 2 cups water (ideally, spring water)
- Half a handful of assorted nuts and seeds

- Ground cloves to taste

Instructions

1. First make the quinoa by following the instructions on the package.
2. Next, drain the quinoa, then pour it into a saucepan. Add the cloves and cayenne. Combine everything.
3. Add the milk and grated lime. Optionally, add grated apple.
4. Top with seeds and nuts. Serve.

PECAN, COCONUT & OATMEAL

Ingredients

- Half a cup of coconut or almond milk
- One tablespoon of coconut flakes

- ¼ teaspoon of pure vanilla extract

- ¼ teaspoon of ground cinnamon

- Two tablespoons of almond flour

- Two tablespoons of hemp hearts

- Two teaspoons of chia seeds

- One tablespoon of flax meal

- One tablespoon of pecans, toasted and chopped

Instructions

1. Combine the chia seeds, flax meal, almond flour, cinnamon, vanilla, hemp hearts, and milk in a small pot. Cook over low heat, stirring occasionally until the mixture becomes thick. This should take about 5 minutes.

2. Spoon everything into a bowl or dish and top with coconut flakes and pecans. Serve immediately.

SPICY KALE

Ingredient

- ¼ cup red pepper, diced
- ¼ tsp sea salt
- 1 tsp red pepper, crushed
- ¼ cup diced onion
- 1 cup kale leaves, chopped
- 2 tbsp grapeseed oil

Instructions

1. Start by heating the grapeseed oil in a pan. Once the oil gets hot, add the diced onion and pepper and saute for about two to three minutes. Next, season with salt.
2. Lower the heat. Then pour in the kale leaves. Cover the pan and simmer for about 5 minutes.
3. Remove the cover and add in the crushed pepper. Stir well, then cover again. Let it cool for about 4 minutes. Serve!

ALKALINE MILLET

Ingredients

- 2 ½ cups water
- 1 cup millet
- ½ tsp sea salt

Instructions

1. First thing is to saute the millet until golden brown. Then add water and salt.
2. Bring the mixture to a boil then simmer for about 30 minutes or until the water is absorbed.
3. Remove from heat and allow to cool with the lid still on. Serve!

AVOCADO & MUNG BEAN SPROUTS SALAD

Ingredients

- Sea salt to taste
- 1 to 2 avocados, diced
- One lime, juiced
- One cup of mung bean sprouts
- Fresh basil
- 1 to 2 tomatoes, cubed
- ¼ cup of olive oil

Instructions

1. Combine all the ingredients in a small bowl. Mix well and serve.

TROPICAL GAZPACHO

Ingredients

- 1½ cups of organic tomato juice
- Salt and pepper
- Tabasco (optional, optional)
- Half a cup of cucumber (peeled, seeded, and chopped)
- Orange ball pepper (half cup, chopped)
- Half small red onion (peeled and chopped)
- Chopped mango (one cup)
- Chopped papaya (one cup)
- Chopped pineapple (half cup)
- Minced cilantro (⅛ cup, fresh)

Directions

1. Put all the ingredients in a blender. Puree them, then transfer to a large bowl and season to taste.
2. Put it in a refrigerator to get cold. Serve and enjoy!

MUESLI WITH NUTS & DRIED FRUIT

Ingredients

- Muesli cereal (half cup)
- Raisins (one tablespoon)
- Half cup of almond milk (you can substitute with low-fat rice or brown rice)
- One teaspoon of almonds (sliced or slivered)
- Walnuts (one teaspoon, chopped)
- Dried berries (one tablespoon, mixed)

Directions

1. Pour the milk and cereal into a bowl to mix them. Add more milk if it's too thick.
2. Use the raisins, walnuts, almonds, and berries as toppings. Serve ASAP.

GINGER TEA

Ingredients

- 2 sprigs dill weed
- 2 tbsp fresh lime juice
- 4 cups spring water
- A pinch of cayenne
- One thumb of fresh ginger root (make sure it's organic; you can also substitute with powder garlic)
- Raw agave to taste (optional)

Instructions

1. Start by boiling the water.
2. Next, peel and chop the ginger root. Then add it to the pot of boiling water followed by the weed.
3. Cook for about 5 minutes, then strain the tea into a glass jar or bowl. Add the lime juice and stir. Finally, add the cayenne and agave. Stir again.
4. Serve either hot or cold.

ALKALINE SALAD

Ingredients

- 4 cups of greens (e.g dandelion, arugula, watercress, etc.)
- 3-4 key limes
- ¼ cup walnuts
- 1 cup cherry tomatoes
- 1 tbsp raw sesame tahini butter
- ¼ cup herb (such as dill or sweet basil)
- Sea salt and cayenne pepper to taste

Instructions

1. Squeeze out the juice from the lime.
2. In a tub, combine the squeezed juice, tahini butter, salt and pepper.
3. Half the tomatoes. In a larger tube, combine the tomatoes, herbs, greens, and the tahini mixture. Mix well and serve.

HYDRATION SMOOTHIE

Ingredients

- ¼ seeded cucumber
- ½ cup soft jelly coconut water
- ½ cup raspberries
- 1 cup watermelon
- 1 key lime, juiced

Instructions

1. First, peel and core the cucumber, then cut it into smaller pieces.
2. Add the cut cucumber to a blender followed by the other ingredients. Blend everything until smooth. Enjoy!

CHAI CHAI DRINK

Ingredients

- One banana
- One cup water
- Half a cup coconut milk
- ¼ tsp ground cinnamon
- ¼ tsp ground ginger
- A pinch of ground cardamom
- One or two medjool dates, pitted
- One tablespoon chia seeds (can be substituted with hemp hearts or ground flax)
- One cup alfalfa sprouts, optional

Instructions

1. Put everything in a blender and puree until smooth.
    You can add more milk or water depending on
    whether you want it thicker or thinner.

STRAWBERRY SMOOTHIE

Ingredients

- Strawberries (two cups, should be about 10 ounces)
- One small banana
- A bunch of fresh spinach (two cups or more)
- One pomegranate
- Flaxseeds (one tablespoon)
- Ice cubes

Directions

1. Remove the seeds in the pomegranate and place
    them in a blender. Add the remaining ingredients.

2. Add ice to fill it up, then set the blender to high
    speed and puree until it's smooth.

3. Pour into two glasses and enjoy. Best served with a
    straw.

ALMOND BUTTER AND WHOLE GRAIN BREAD

Ingredients

- Almond butter (one tablespoon)

- Whole Grain Bread (one slice)

- Half medium pear (peeled, cored, sliced)

- Chopped walnuts (one teaspoon)

Directions

1. Spread the butter over the bread. Then place the
    sliced pears on top.

2. Sprinkle with walnuts. Enjoy!

SOUTHERN ONION SOUP

Ingredients

- Three tablespoons of olive oil

- Two cups sweet onions, thinly sliced (such as Vidalia)

- One dash of nutmeg

- One 10 ½ oz package of soft silken tofu

- Four cups of salted vegetable stock (if stock is not salted, you can add half a teaspoon of salt)

Instructions

1. Start by sautéing the onions and olive oil in a skillet until transparent over medium heat.

2. Pour the vegetable stock into a saucepan and add in the sautéd onions. Cover the saucepan and simmer for 25 to 30 minutes or until the onions become very soft.

3. Remove the saucepan from heat and pour the soup into a blender. Optionally, break a block of soft tofu into smaller pieces and add to the soup in the blender.

4. Now, blend for two to three minutes or until smooth.

5. Finally, transfer the soup in the blender into dishes and garnish with a dash of nutmeg. Serve hot or chilled.

EASY TEFF PORRIDGE

Ingredients

- ½ cup teff grain
- 2 cups of water (ideally, spring water)
- A pinch of salt
- Blueberries and agave nectar to taste

Ingredients

1. Pour the water into a saucepan and bring to a boil. Then add the salt and teff grain. Stir thoroughly.

2. Reduce the heat to low heat and simmer for 15 minutes with the lid on.

3. Serve with blueberries and agave as toppings.

EASY FRUIT SALAD

Ingredients

- One pint of fresh strawberries, sliced without stems
- One pint of fresh blueberries
- Two cups of grapes
- One ripe pear, cored and diced
- Two tablespoons of date syrup, optional
- ¼ tsp ground cinnamon

Instructions

1. Combine all the ingredients in a bowl. Stir to mix well.

2. Keep in the refrigerator and serve chill.

HERBERT HUMMUS

Ingredients

- ¼ cup of chives, chopped
- Half a cup of fresh tarragon leaves, blanched with light packing
- Two garlic cloves
- One cup of fresh basil leaves, blanched with light packing
- Four cups of garbanzo beans, cooked
- Freshly squeezed juice from one lemon
- One cup of vegetable broth
- Half a cup of fresh flat parsley leaves
- Two tablespoons of sesame seeds, toasted

Instructions

1. Start by dabbing the basil leaves and tarragon until dry. Then cut into smaller sizes and add to a blender.
2. Next, also add the lemon juice, beans, sesame seeds, garlic, lemon juice, and vegetable broth to the blender. Blend until smooth and creamy.

Add chives and stir. Enjoy.

ELECTRIC SALAD

Ingredients

- Olive oil
- 1 cup cherry tomatoes
- 1 cup kale, chopped
- 2 red onions
- 3 Jalapenos

- A handful of romaine lettuce

- Juice from 1 lime

- 1 orange pepper

- 1 yellow pepper

Directions

1. Wash and rinse the ingredients. After drying, cut into smaller bite-sized pieces.

2. Put everything in a bowl, then drizzle with the olive oil and lemon juice. Enjoy!

EASY VEGETABLE BROTH

Ingredients

- Eight cups of water

- Three ribs of celery, chopped

- Five cloves of garlic, minced

- Three carrots, chopped
- Two bay leaves
- Two to three cups of vegetable scraps, frozen
- Two large onions, chopped
- A few sprigs of thyme
- A few sprigs of parsley
- One tablespoon of olive oil
- Salt and pepper to taste

Instructions

1. Start by heating the olive oil in a large stockpot or Dutch oven over medium heat.
2. Once the oil is hot, add in the onions, carrots, and celery and cook until softened. This should take about 5 minutes. Make sure to stir frequently.
3. Next, add the water and the remaining ingredients - bay leaves, thyme, parsley, and frozen vegetable scraps. Reduce the stove to low heat and simmer for about 45 minutes with the pot partially covered.

4. Now, pour the broth through a fine mesh strainer into another large pot or bowl. You can discard the solids.

5. Allow the broth to cool, then pour it into freezer bags or airtight containers and keep in the freezer until you're ready to use it.

VEGETABLE STOCK

Ingredients

- Fresh thyme (one small bunch)
- Four medium-sized carrots, chopped
- A handful of fresh parsley
- One garlic bulb, halved
- Two medium-sized onions, halved
- One to two medium-sized celery stalks, chopped
- Three bay leaves

- 10-12 cups of filtered water

- 2 teaspoons of sea salt

- 1 teaspoon of black peppercorns

- Leek or fennel tops, chopped (I would use 1-2 cups but you can use more or lesser)

Instructions

1. In a large pot, combine the pepper, salt, leek tops, onions, carrots, celery, garlic, parsley, baly leaves, thyme and water, and place over high heat to boil.

2. Lower the heat and simmer for one hour with the cover of the pot still on.

3. Strain into a bowl and discard the vegetables.

FRUIT PUNCH

Ingredients

- One and half cups of natural orange juice

- Four cups of natural cranberry juice

- One and half cups of pineapple juice

- Three cups of ginger ale, chilled

- ¼ cup lime juice

- Sliced fruit for serving

Instructions

1. Stir all the juice together in a large pitcher- orange juice, pineapple juice, lime juice and cranberry juice.
2. Chill overnight or at least four hours before serving. The ginger ale and sliced fruit can be added before serving.

GRANOLA

Ingredients

- Honey (¼ cup)

- Grapeseed oil (¼ cup)

- Cinnamon (two teaspoons)

- Almond extract (one teaspoon)

- Orange extract (one teaspoon)

- Rolled oats (three and half cups)

- Slivered almonds (¼ cup)

- Walnuts (¼ cup, chopped)

Directions

1. Preheat the oven. The temperature should be 350 degrees Fahrenheit.

2. Pour the honey into a bowl, then add all the extracts, oil, and spices.

3. Add the nuts and oats and stir well.

4. Now, spread the mixture over a greased cookie sheet. Bake for ten minutes, then stir and continue to bake for another 10 minutes or until the mixture turns golden brown.

5. Let it cool, then you can break it apart. Put into a container for storage. The container should be airtight. Enjoy!

6. This can be topped with fruits and enjoyed with your favorite plant-based milk drink such as low-fat soy milk or almond oil.
7. To make things more interesting, you can add a teaspoon of freshly grounded flaxseeds to each serving.

CHAMOMILE TEA

What You Need

- Chamomile flower (you need a handful)
- Spring water (one cup)

How to Make It

1. Pour the water into a tea kettle, then add the flowers.
2. Heat for five minutes or until it boils. Take it away from the heat, cover it, and leave for extra ten minutes.

3. Drain the tea and serve!

CHUNKY MONKEY SMOOTHIE

Ingredients

- One cup of unsweetened almond milk (use same amount of water if you don't have almond milk)
- One tablespoon of unsweetened cocoa
- Half a cup of medjool dates, pitted and chopped
- Two medium bananas, peeled and cut into chunks
- One table of peanut butter (optional)

Instructions

1. Add all the ingredients to a blender and blend until creamy. Feel free to add more milk to make it more creamy. Enjoy.

Conclusion

To conclude, if you're dealing with POTS, I want you to know that you're not alone. While this can be frustrating and interfere with your daily life, with the right diet and a little bit of physical activity, you can find relief.

The good news is that, in most cases, POTS symptoms can clear up on their own, even though it might take a while.